A Call To Christian Veganism

By Ryan Hicks

Version 1.1

Notice:

No part of this book may be reproduced or transmitted in any form or by any means, electronic or mechanical, including photocopying, recording or by any information storage and retrieval system, without written permission from the author.

Disclaimer:

The author has made every effort to ensure the accuracy of the information within this book was correct at time of publication. The author does not assume and hereby disclaims any liability to any party for any loss, damage, or disruption caused by errors or omissions, whether such errors or omissions result from accident, negligence, or any other cause.

For discussion about the
topics raised in this book,
please visit:
ChristianVeganism.com

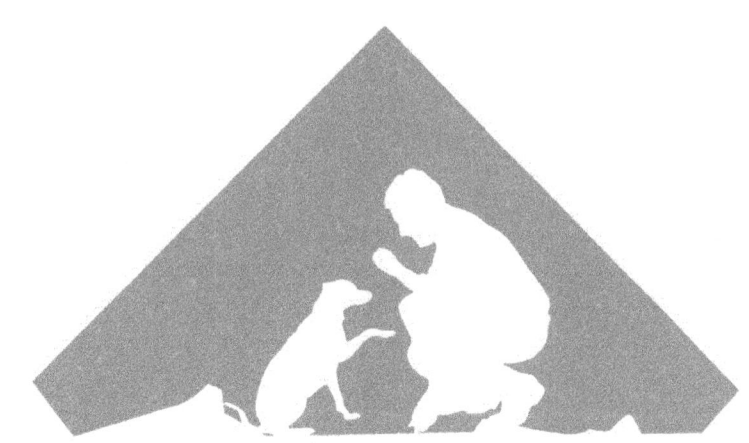

ChristianVeganism.com

TABLE OF CONTENTS

Introduction

This book is meant to give a concise summary of the rationale behind Christian veganism. Much of modern Christendom, just like pre-reformation Christendom, is mired in error and blindness. This short book does not intend to answer all the common objections professing Christians might have to veganism. I have dealt with all those questions and passages of Scripture in my over 400-page book titled "Why Every Christian Should Be A Vegan," which you can get at https://www.ChristianVeganism.com.

I will reference my book "Why Every Christian Should Be A Vegan" throughout this book to highlight the subjects that you might want to study further which are dealt with in that book. Since that book is over 400 pages long, I cannot duplicate the topics in it here, because the purpose of this book is to be very succinct and hopefully convincing to those who are feeling a stirring in their souls about Christian veganism. You would do well also to read "Why Every Christian Should Be A Vegan" if you believe that you need all your major objections answered or if you would like a more in-depth approach to this topic.

This book is NOT about a mere difference of opinion or a matter of personal dietary choice. The issue of veganism directly relates to your personal morality, Christian ethics, and whether you are living your life as best you can to honor God. Apologist vegans get caught up in trivializing the importance of veganism amongst Christians and settle for double-mindedness like being a flexitarian or vegetarian. Veganism is far more than a simple dietary choice; it is a lifestyle of compassion, mercy, and peace towards the other sentient beings we share the planet with: the animals.

I must be clear that I did not come from a vegan household or even a vegetarian one. I was raised on the standard American diet that was very high in animal products and very low in fruits and vegetables. I came to veganism from a conviction by the Spirit of God in my inner man that I was engaging in violence every time I ate the flesh of an animal or partook of the products of their exploitation and suffering, such as eggs or milk (none of which had been intended for human consumption). I did not become a vegan for health reasons, even though it is the best diet for your health. I also did not become a vegan to save the environment, even though veganism is the best way to be a good steward of the planet God has given us.

It is my prayer that you will genuinely consider what I have written in this book and that you will also read my in-depth book on Christian veganism, "Why Every Christian Should Be A Vegan." I do believe that the Church of Jesus Christ is at the point of reawakening to the original form of Christianity which did not partake of animal flesh and sought to make earth as much like heaven as they possibly could.

Job 5:22-24

22 At destruction and famine thou shalt laugh: neither shalt thou be afraid of the beasts of the earth.

23 For thou shalt be in league with the stones of the field: and the beasts of the field shall be at peace with thee.

24 And thou shalt know that thy tabernacle *shall be* in peace; and thou shalt visit thy habitation, and shalt not sin.

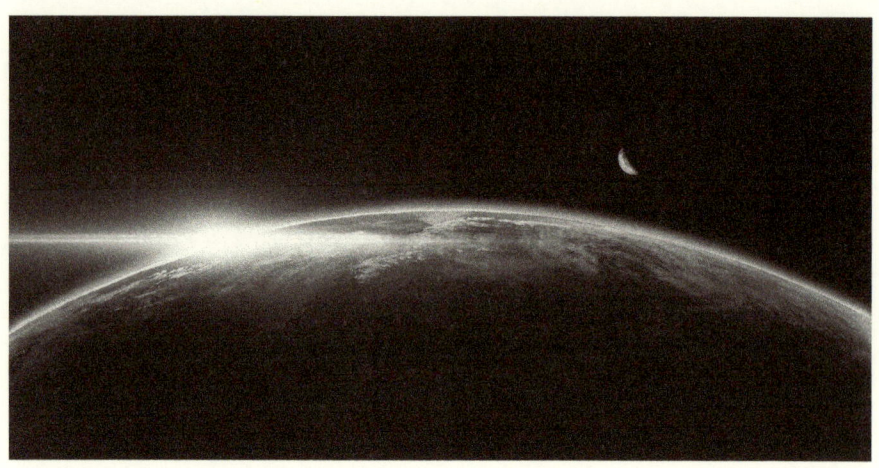

Chapter 1
In The Beginning

Genesis 1:1
1 In the beginning God created the heaven and the earth.

There is little debate amongst believers that the original creation template for humans and animals was to be a vegan world of peace and love, and yet, somehow, humans have adopted this fallen idea that animals were created and currently exist only for them to use, abuse, and even eat. The actual information given about humans and animals in the Scripture tells a very different story from the one that most seem to have embraced.

Genesis 2:18-20
18 And the LORD God said, *It is* not good that the man should be alone; I will make him an help meet for him.
19 And out of the ground the LORD God formed every beast of the field, and every fowl of the air; and brought *them* unto Adam to see what

he would call them: and whatsoever Adam called every living creature, that *was* the name thereof.

20 And Adam gave names to all cattle, and to the fowl of the air, and to every beast of the field; but for Adam there was not found an help meet for him.

Carefully notice the first part of this passage of Scripture. God says that it is not good for man to be alone, and then what does He do in response to this? He creates animals! Animals were created to be companions with man, rather than be beings that exist only for the utility, entertainment, or food for man. They were designed to be friends, companions, and fellow earth-dwellers. So deep was this companionship between man and animal that Adam even gave the animals their names, like a parent would name their children.

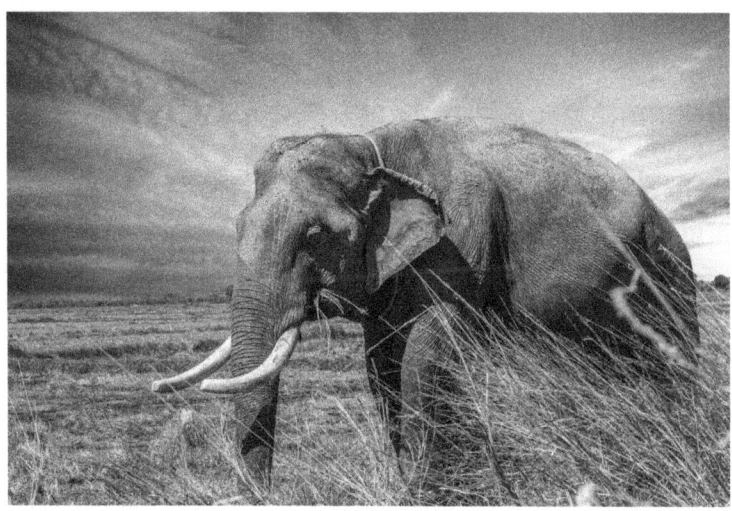

Genesis 2:21-23

21 And the LORD God caused a deep sleep to fall upon Adam, and he slept: and he took one

of his ribs, and closed up the flesh instead thereof;

22 And the rib, which the LORD God had taken from man, made he a woman, and brought her unto the man.

23 And Adam said, This *is* now bone of my bones, and flesh of my flesh: she shall be called Woman, because she was taken out of Man.

God saw that the animals were not enough companionship for Adam and that he needed someone like himself: another human. The fact that Adam needed someone more like him for companionship did not discount the companionship of animals, nor did it relegate animals to the position of being mistreated, abused, or eaten. They were still the companions of humanity, and Adam and Eve were given dominion over animals:

Genesis 1:26-28

26 And God said, Let us make man in our image, after our likeness: and let them have dominion over the fish of the sea, and over the fowl of the air, and over the cattle, and over all the earth, and over every creeping thing that creepeth upon the earth.

27 So God created man in his *own* image, in the image of God created he him; male and female created he them.

28 And God blessed them, and God said unto them, Be fruitful, and multiply, and replenish the earth, and subdue it: and have dominion over the fish of the sea, and over the fowl of the air, and over every living thing that moveth upon the earth.

This passage of Scripture establishes a critical point

that is often misunderstood. Frequently people will argue for cruelty and mercilessness towards animals because Adam and Eve were given dominion over them. This idea of dominion is a complete perversion of the compassionate dominion that God gave humanity. The dominion given to humanity over animals mentioned in these verses is that of stewardship. It is the same dominion that a parent has over their child. It is not God granting humans a reign of tyranny over the earth.

> **Genesis 1:29-30**
> **29** And God said, Behold, I have given you every herb bearing seed, which *is* upon the face of all the earth, and every tree, in the which *is* the fruit of a tree yielding seed; to you it shall be for meat.
> **30** And to every beast of the earth, and to every fowl of the air, and to every thing that creepeth upon the earth, wherein *there is* life, *I have given* every green herb for meat: and it was so.

The original diet for humans and animals was plant-based. Humans and animals were to live together in peace, eating from the plants that God created for them to eat. The perversion of killing another being and eating their flesh was never a part of this original plan. That was an evil that came as a result of sin entering the world.

What is important to note is that even after Adam and Eve brought sin into the world, God still held them to a vegan diet:

> **Genesis 3:17-19**
> **17** And unto Adam he said, Because thou hast

hearkened unto the voice of thy wife, and hast eaten of the tree, of which I commanded thee, saying, Thou shalt not eat of it: cursed *is* the ground for thy sake; in sorrow shalt thou eat *of* it all the days of thy life;

18 Thorns also and thistles shall it bring forth to thee; and thou shalt eat the herb of the field;

19 In the sweat of thy face shalt thou eat bread, till thou return unto the ground; for out of it wast thou taken: for dust thou *art,* and unto dust shalt thou return.

No mention was ever made here of humans turning from grace toward the great evil of killing their fellow sentient beings and eating them. Even after sin came into the world, it was still understood that the diet for humanity was plant-based.

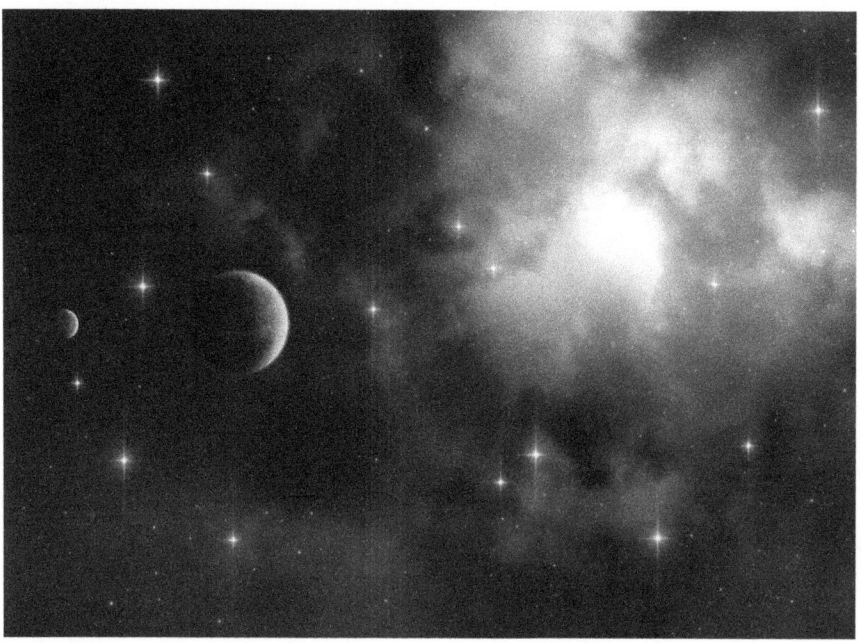

Chapter 2
In The Future

Isaiah 11:6-9

6 The wolf also shall dwell with the lamb, and the leopard shall lie down with the kid; and the calf and the young lion and the fatling together; and a little child shall lead them.

7 And the cow and the bear shall feed; their young ones shall lie down together: and the lion shall eat straw like the ox.

8 And the sucking child shall play on the hole of the asp, and the weaned child shall put his hand on the cockatrice' den.

9 They shall not hurt nor destroy in all my holy mountain: for the earth shall be full of the knowledge of the LORD, as the waters cover the sea.

We have seen that God's original plan for humans and animals was that of companionship. As the compassionate rulers of the planet, humans were to have an almost parental role over animals to protect them and seek their betterment. In eternity's future, we also see that God restores the planet to this original order of compassion and companionship. This passage in Isaiah 11 illustrates so profoundly that former predators and prey are now companions, and little children can safely lead animals in peace that were dangerous in previous times.

It is worth noting the last verse in the above passage of Scripture. When the earth is full of the knowledge of the LORD, what then happens? Humanity does not go to war, does not harm each other, and does not harm animals. When humans get the true knowledge of God in their hearts, then they naturally depart from causing harm. Harm is a depraved monument to the fallen world, but peace, love, and compassion are the reigning principles of the restored earth in eternity's future.

> **Ezekiel 34:25-26**
> **25** And I will make with them a covenant of peace, and will cause the evil beasts to cease out of the land: and they shall dwell safely in the wilderness, and sleep in the woods.
> **26** And I will make them and the places round about my hill a blessing; and I will cause the shower to come down in his season; there shall be showers of blessing.

> **Hosea 2:18**
> **18** And in that day will I make a covenant for them with the beasts of the field, and with the fowls of heaven, and *with* the creeping things of

the ground: and I will break the bow and the sword and the battle out of the earth, and will make them to lie down safely.

It is essential to see how God interacts with both humans and animals. He makes covenants with both alike. Animals are not merely things; they are sentient beings who God makes covenants with and loves. To think that a human would call themselves a lover of God while destroying and eating one of God's covenant partners is perversion in the highest degree; and yet, people do this day in and day out, never seeming to see or even care about God's love for His creation.

I go in-depth into all the covenants that God has made with animals and the state of animals as beings with souls (sentient beings) in Chapter 47, "God's Covenant With Animals" and Chapter 46, "Animals Have Immortal Souls" of my book "Why Every Christian Should Be A Vegan," which is available at https://www.ChristianVeganism.com.

Isaiah 65:25
25 The wolf and the lamb shall feed together, and the lion shall eat straw like the bullock: and dust *shall be* the serpent's meat. They shall not hurt nor destroy in all my holy mountain, saith the LORD.

Once again, we see that God's eternal plan for man and animals is that we are restored to His original plan of peace and doing no harm. It is also important to see that animals will be restored to their original plant-based diet so that the wolf and lamb feed together and the lion eats straw like the bullock.

What you need to ask yourself is a few things. If God's original plan for humans was for them to be compassionate and do no harm (to other humans or animals) and His eternal plan is to restore humans and animals fully back to this original peaceable kingdom, then why would you choose to not enact such a peaceable kingdom in your heart right now? How could you claim to want to do God's will, while rejecting His eternal will of peace and harmlessness?

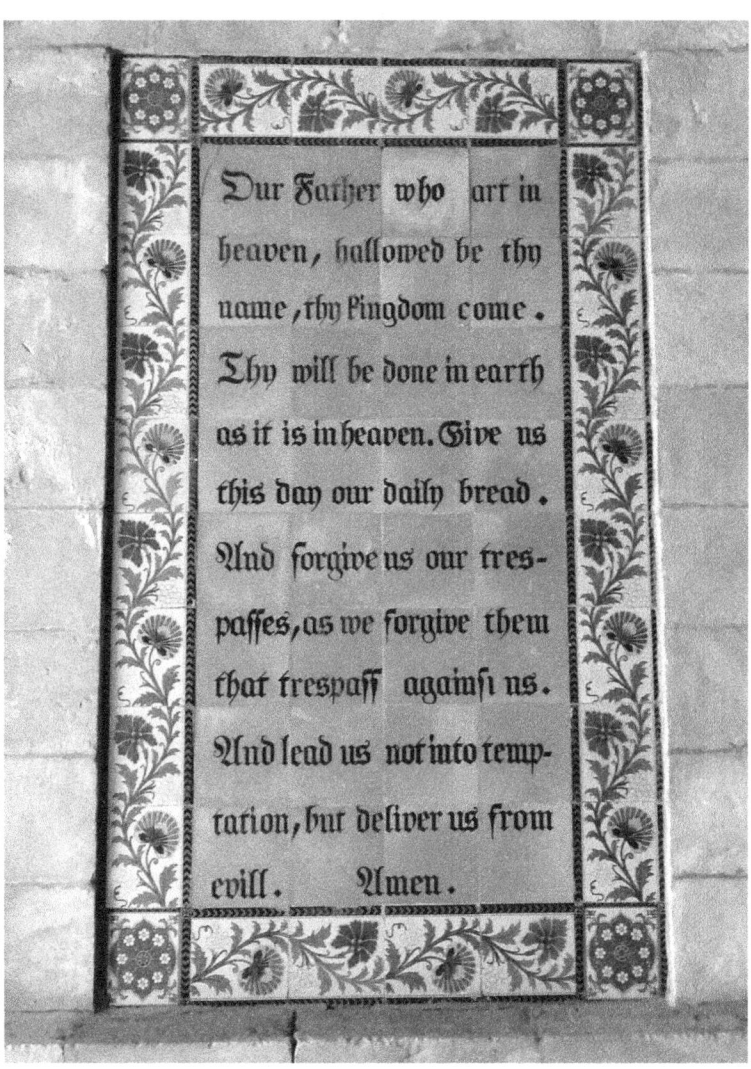

Chapter 3
The Lord's Prayer

Matthew 6:9-13 records Jesus giving what is commonly known as "The Lord's Prayer:"

Our Father which art in heaven, Hallowed be thy name. Thy kingdom come. Thy will be done in earth, as *it is* in heaven. Give us this day our daily bread. And forgive us our debts, as we forgive our debtors. And lead us not into temptation, but deliver us from evil: For thine is the kingdom, and the power, and the glory, for ever. Amen.

The Lord's prayer is one of the most quoted prayers in human history. While many millions may pray this prayer daily, few truly mean a word of it, as their actions so plainly testify. People repeat this prayer as a vain repetition and then continue apathetically eating animals, eating the eggs and milk of animals, and using animals for products, entertainment, or cruelty, never making the words of their prayer their heartfelt desire. They could not partake of any of these things if they sincerely took the Lord's prayer seriously and intended to enact it in their lives each day. Let us look at the Lord's prayer and notice one of the powerful truths that very few seem to be able to see in it:

> **Matthew 6:9-13**
> **9** After this manner therefore pray ye: Our Father which art in heaven, Hallowed be thy name.
> **10** Thy kingdom come. Thy will be done in earth, as *it is* in heaven.
> **11** Give us this day our daily bread.
> **12** And forgive us our debts, as we forgive our debtors.
> **13** And lead us not into temptation, but deliver us from evil: For thine is the kingdom, and the power, and the glory, for ever. Amen.

Notice verse 10, which says, "Thy will be done in

earth, as it is in heaven." I want you to stop reading this book for a few minutes and deeply ponder that sentence.

The Lord teaches in this prayer that your earnest desire is to be for God's will to be done on earth, "as it is in heaven." This truth is paramount because we know that there is no harm, suffering, or death in heaven. How can a person pray this prayer in good conscience if they promptly deny this fundamental truth by rejecting God's will completely and eating animals or causing them harm?

Many may even realize this truth and stop eating animal flesh or wearing things like leather or fur, but few realize that there is even more cruelty in the egg and dairy industries, which I deal with in-depth in Chapter 7, "Eggs And Dairy Must Be Humane, Right?" of my book "Why Every Christian Should Be A Vegan." The cruelty and suffering caused by the egg and dairy industries may come as a shock to you, but it is the tragic reality of the experience animals are forced to endure only because people will not give up their fleshly lust for eggs, dairy, and animal flesh.

Some will appeal to futility and argue that we cannot perfectly implement God's will on earth, so why even try? Such a mindset of apathy is not the mindset of a person who is after God's own heart. Even if your choice to do the right thing has little impact in this world, you should still always choose to do the right thing. Can you imagine this mindset when abolitionist Christians spoke out against human slavery? There could still be slavery in developed places like the United States if good people had just sat back and said that it was futile to even try to make a change. Even if you are the only person doing the right thing, you should still be that one to do it, because that should be your character and nature as a child of God.

As you can see, this is where veganism becomes a real matter of the heart. As you grow in grace, you should be seeking each day to implement God's will in your life more perfectly. Veganism is a straightforward way that you can be at peace with animals and not be causing them any harm (or in the very least, your choice to become a vegan will limit the harm as much as possible).

There are many weak excuses that people come up with when they are battling against their conscience and the leading of the Spirit calling them to become vegans. Veganism is a moral issue, so there is no need for "baby steps" or "transitioning over to veganism." Such would be like an abusive husband saying that he was going to transition over to being a loving husband by only beating his wife six days a week instead of seven. Yes, such would be less evil, but it is still evil. Your goal should be to strive to enact God's perfect will in your life wherein it is at all possible. You should not be trying to find ways to half-heartedly transition to doing what is right or merely pay lip service to having integrity of heart.

"Transitioning" to veganism is merely an excuse that people make because they want to keep partaking in something which they now realize to be harmful and contrary to their souls. You are not honoring God when you just cut out eating "meat" from your diet because you still cause the death and torture of animals through the eggs and dairy you consume, the clothing you wear, and the products you use. Yes, you may be causing less harm, but you are still refusing to really honor God with your life. Give up such feeble and lukewarm approaches to life and choose to do what is right.

> **Revelation 3:15-16**
> **15** I know thy works, that thou art neither cold nor hot: I would thou wert cold or hot.
> **16** So then because thou art lukewarm, and neither cold nor hot, I will spue thee out of my mouth.

I believe that the Spirit of Grace is calling many who have read this far to choose to have a vegan diet _and_ lifestyle. Surely, you must now see the importance of honoring God with your life and want to be aligned with His perfect will?

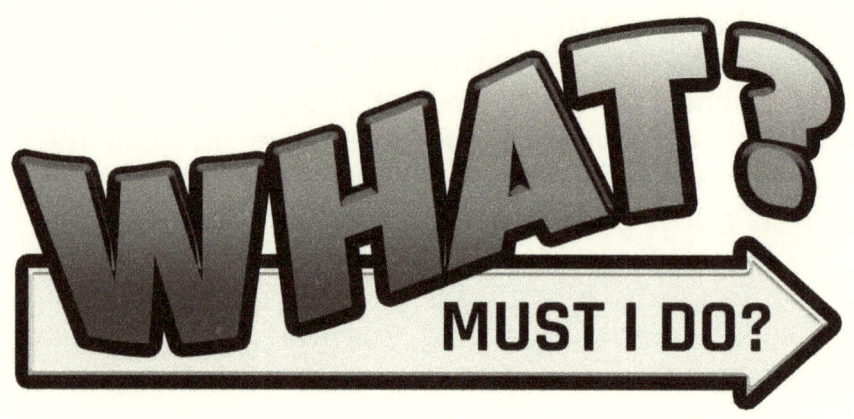

Chapter 4
What Must I Do?

1 Thessalonians 5:22
22 Abstain from all appearance of evil.

The animal agriculture industry is universally awash in ceaseless evil. I deal with some of the practices of the animal agriculture industry, including the feigned "humane family farms," that are widely accepted in my book "Why Every Christian Should Be A Vegan." Suffice it to say, the commonly accepted "humane" practices in this industry are still genuinely evil, and something in which few professing Christians would want to be associated. There are readily available documentaries such as Earthlings and Dominion which document the momentous evil that occurs to get people their meat, dairy, eggs, fur, leather, and other animal-sourced products.

1 Corinthians 10:31-33
31 Whether therefore ye eat, or drink, or whatsoever ye do, do all to the glory of God.
32 Give none offence, neither to the Jews, nor to the Gentiles, nor to the church of God:

33 Even as I please all *men* in all *things,* not seeking mine own profit, but the *profit* of many, that they may be saved.

No self-proclaimed omnivore (i.e. necrovore[1]) cares if you are vegan and eat a plant-based diet, but many compassionate people will care and be offended by your choice to eat animal flesh, dairy, and eggs. How can you be eating or drinking to the glory of God when you choose to purposely offend people from Christ by engaging in a diet and lifestyle that is contrary to the perfect will of God?

> **Romans 14:15-17**
> **15** But if thy brother be grieved with *thy* meat, now walkest thou not charitably. Destroy not him with thy meat, for whom Christ died.
> **16** Let not then your good be evil spoken of:
> **17** For the kingdom of God is not meat and drink; but righteousness, and peace, and joy in the Holy Ghost.

Besides the obvious point of wanting to best honor God by implanting as much of His perfect will in our lives as we can, another vital point is that eating animals, using them for products or entertainment,

---

[1] A necrovore human is a person that eats decaying flesh (erroneously referred to as an omnivore human). Humans are not carnivorous, as they do not eat the fresh flesh of their prey. They eat the decaying and putrefying flesh of dead animals, generally that other people killed. Even hunters do not eat the freshly killed flesh. Animal flesh in stores may be months old and have undergone bleaching, dying, or other processing to make it look "fresh" and cover up the decomposition of the decaying flesh.

and other such forms of abuse also cause harm to compassionate believers who are aligned with God and take joy in His animals. You grieve your brother who loves God and His creation when you choose a lifestyle of harm, death, and treachery over the compassionate vegan lifestyle that is God's eternal will for humanity and animals alike.

It is a direct sin against Christ to continue in a non-vegan lifestyle that causes harm to animals, the planet, and pure-hearted believers (1 Corinthians 8:12). It also causes non-believers who have compassion for animals to reject Christ because they view Christians as evil people who are violent and cruel towards animals (which is the opposite of what an authentic Christian is). The saddest part is that the only reason for all this harm and needless offense that the animal flesh and animal-sourced product imbiber causes is due to their fleshly desire for specific tastes that they have been culturally programmed to enjoy. You will see later in this book that these tastes have been replicated and improved in compassionate plant-based substitutes, so the "I can't help that I have the taste for flesh" argument is invalid.

Can you honestly stand before God and say that your steak was more important than the eternal soul of one who rejected Christ because they saw your ways as evil? Do you want to be the one who puts their tastebuds above love, compassion, and mercy? Do you want to be one who sets the example of compassion, godliness, and honor or one who is caught up in carnality, fleshly lusts, and the traditions of men?

Romans 14:21
21 *It is* good neither to eat flesh, nor to drink

wine, nor *any thing* whereby thy brother stumbleth, or is offended, or is made weak.

Notice that it is plainly stated that it is good to neither drink wine nor eat flesh. If something you are doing is unnecessarily causing harm to others, then it is good not to do it. Merely continuing forward in the destructive behavior because you like the taste of something is fleshly, evil, and an affront to Christ.

> **James 4:17**
> 17 Therefore to him that knoweth to do good, and doeth *it* not, to him it is sin.

I have had professing Christians tell me that they know how horrible it is to eat animals, eat eggs, or drink milk, and yet they continue to do so. They will say things like, "I can't give up bacon," or "I do not know what I would do without cheese." No believer should be in bondage to any lust of the flesh like this. Being controlled or ruled by certain foods is the sign of being out of control and undisciplined. It is more akin to those mentioned in the Scripture "whose God *is their* belly, and *whose* glory *is* in their shame, who mind earthly things" (Philippians 3:19).

> **Romans 16:18**
> 18 For they that are such serve not our Lord Jesus Christ, but their own belly; and by good words and fair speeches deceive the hearts of the simple.

If you find yourself considering what you will be giving up by going vegan, I would hope that you realize that for all animal-sourced products you may currently use, from leather to meat to milk to cheese to eggs, there are higher quality plant-based substitutes and replacements that taste or work as good or better than the animal-sourced product.

In Chapter 61, "I Should Go Vegan, But I Love The Taste Of "Meat!" in my book, "Why Every Christian Should Be A Vegan," I list numerous examples of vegan meat, egg, and dairy substitutes winning non-vegan food tasting competitions. It may seem cute to repeat old, outdated sayings about how vegan meat substitutes "taste like cardboard" or "are like eating the soles of shoes" but repeating these things only reveals a woeful ignorance of the current reality and a really tragic choice to foolishly "speak evil of those things which they know not" (Jude 10).

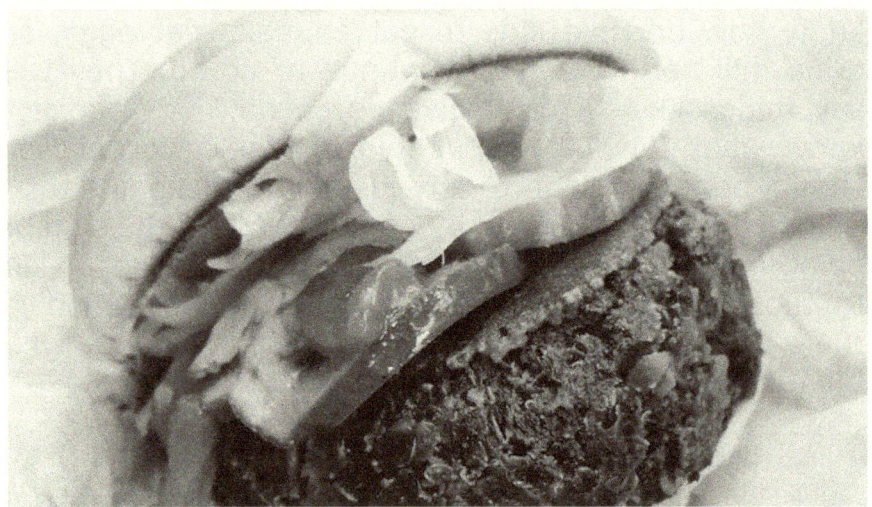
Image source: Instagram User @nycbynyc

The burger above is 100% plant-based. It is called the Superiority Burger and was determined to be the best burger of the year by non-vegans.

The image below is of one of the many plant-based seafood alternatives. This one is called Tuno and is a vegan tuna substitute that tastes just like tuna, with no animals having to suffer for the flavor. You can learn more about this delicious plant-based tuna at https://ChristianVeganism.com/links/tuna

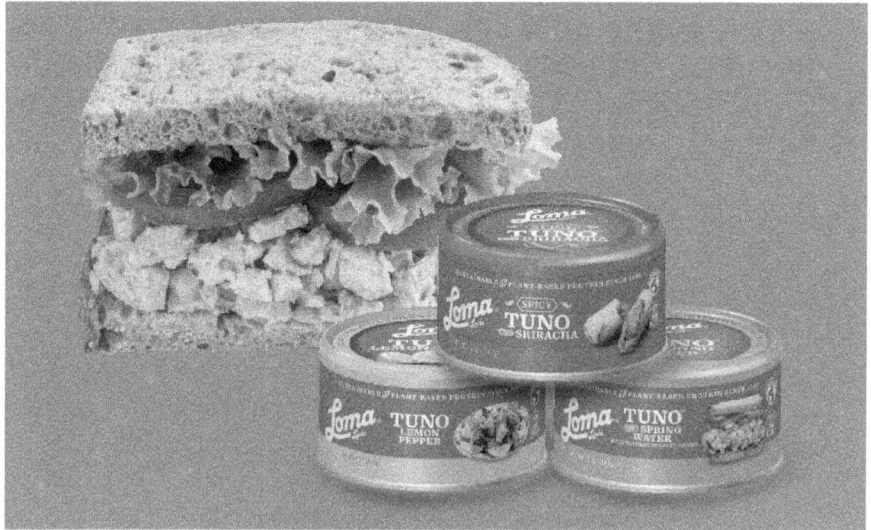

Image source: Tuno

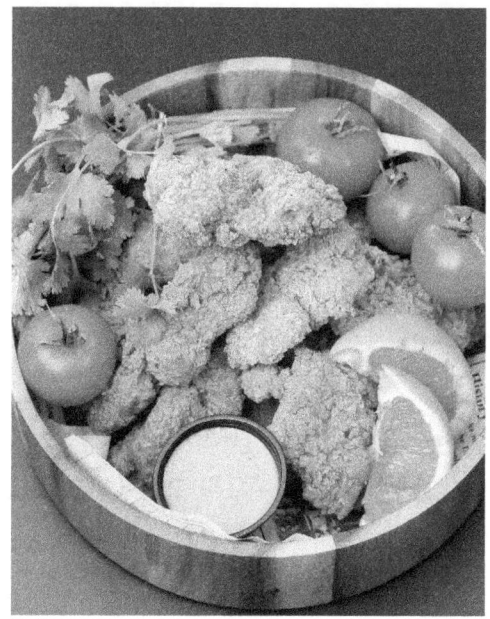

Image source: Instagram Atlas.Monroe

The Cajun plant-based fried "chicken" shown in the previous picture was determined to be the best at the National Fried Chicken Festival in New Orleans. It was the only vegan offering in the entire festival! The "vegan catering company Atlas Monroe's plant-based Cajun Fried Chicken and Waffles were declared "the best" by Time's EXTRA CRISPY editor, and one of the event's judges, Ryan Grim." (Source: https://www.livekindly.co/vegan-fried-chicken-vendor-atlas-monroe/)

Just this one vegan food company, Atlas Monroe, offers many plant-based products like:

➢ ORGANIC VEGAN CAJUN SOUTHERN FRIED CHICKEN - BREAST/THIGH SIZED PIECES

➢ ORGANIC VEGAN CURED BACON

➢ ORGANIC VEGAN APPLE WOOD FIRED RIBS

➢ ORGANIC VEGAN DEEP FRIED & STUFFED TURKEY

You can see more about them and their products at https://atlasmonroe.com/orderfoodnow/

Atlas Monroe is just one company that I chose at random (and have no affiliation with), but there are thousands of small vegan food companies in the world, and even many of the largest food companies are offering vegan meat, dairy, and egg substitutes now.

Gone are the days where people claimed they were limited or restricted to bland tastes if they chose to be vegans. There are endless options now and no excuse at all to continue eating and using animal-sourced products. There is just no reason for you not to choose to be a vegan when it is right morally, environmentally, health-wise, and ethically. You have an obligation in Christ to be a light to the world, and one easy way to be a greater light to the world is to become a Christian vegan!

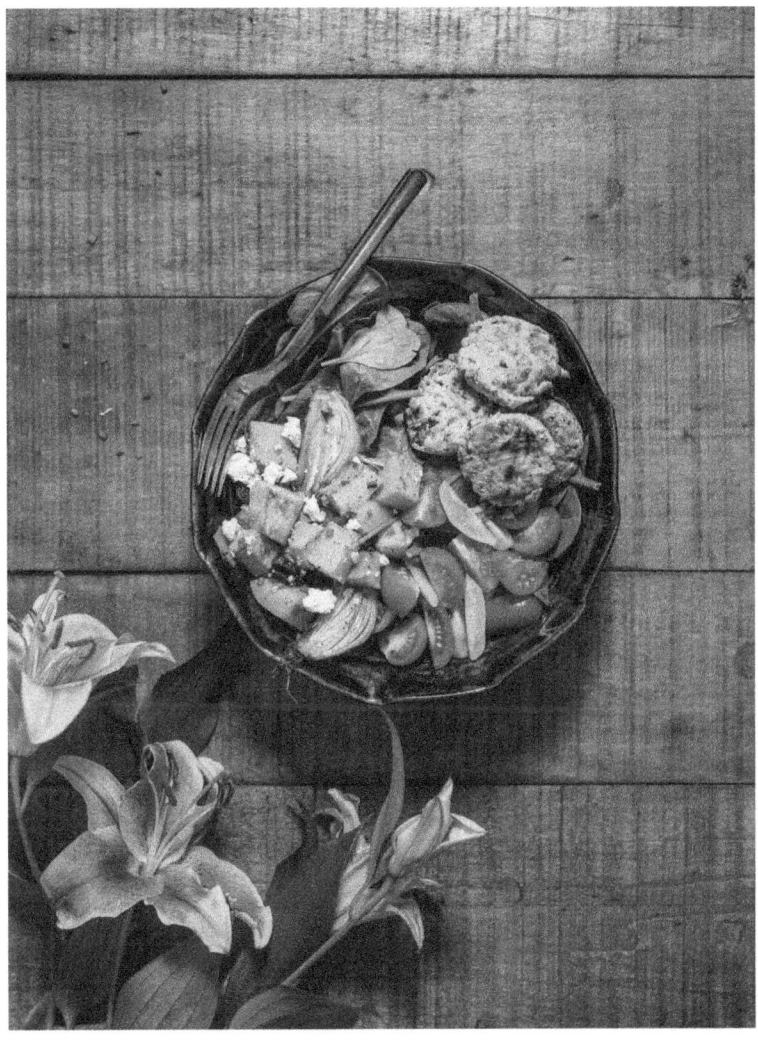

The taste argument against veganism is invalid and

exposes the sad truth that people choose harmful animal-sourced products over plant-based ones for no reason other than apathy and the traditions of men they blindly follow. If they genuinely wanted the best taste, then they would choose the vegan products that are so plenteously available now, since such products far surpass the taste of the animal-sourced versions every single time.

Even amongst the animal flesh products, people do not like the taste by itself. They always must add plant-based spices and sauces to make it edible. Look at one of the most popular animal flesh products: the hamburger. The traditional animal-based burger is loaded with a plant-based bun, vegetables like lettuce and tomatoes, plant-based sauces like ketchup and mustard, etc. Many do not want to face the fact that most of their affinity for animal flesh and animal-sourced products is merely cultural and has nothing to do with them getting the best tasting foods. They must purposely skip the best tasting foods (which happen to be vegan) to continue eating animal-sourced products.

It may be of interest to you to learn that the Apostle Paul plainly states that he is a vegan in the New Testament. Many have gotten lost in his style of argumentation, and erroneously believed that he was against veganism and advocated for carnism, but the opposite is the truth. I deal with this issue in detail in Chapter 32, "Vegans Have Weak Faith?" and Chapter 33, "Paul Says To Eat Flesh?," in my book "Why Every Christian Should Be A Vegan," but it is worth briefly discussing here:

1 Corinthians 8:13
13 Wherefore, if meat make my brother to

offend, I will eat no flesh while the world standeth, lest I make my brother to offend.

Paul took the point of not offending a brother in the Lord to such an extreme that he would never do the thing that could offend them. Even if you wanted to wrongly argue from the position of what God has permitted evil men to do, this verse alone would be enough to convince the Christian to give up their blood lust for animal flesh and all the cruelty involved in animal-sourced products once and for all. Your choice to be non-vegan harms your brethren and offends many from the faith. Your body has zero need for any animal products, and you do not need their skins or fur for clothing. You are literally choosing the most harmful, cruel, and merciless option when you decide against veganism.

Some will argue that they can still "go to heaven" if they are non-vegans, but this is hardly a valid argument for such a tremendously harmful lifestyle of mercilessness. Christians will spend eternity with the Lord, in part, because they have been made new creatures in Christ (2 Corinthians 5:17). You cannot go into eternity with the same evil and defiled heart that follows the lust of the flesh, because Christians have crucified the flesh with the affections and lusts (Galatians 5:24).

Christians are no longer living from this selfish place of just trying to escape hell or punishment for their sins. They are trying to live their lives for God's glory. It is simply untenable to believe that God gets more glory out of you harming animals by eating them, wearing their skin, or using them for products, entertainment, or testing. How can God get glory from you destroying the beings He created for His pleasure

(Revelation 4:11)?

If God intended you to abuse and eat animals, then that is the way He would have created things, but we have seen that His perfect will had humans and animals alike eat plants for food. In God's perfect will humans are caretakers of animals with loving dominion over them like a parent has dominion over their child.

We have also seen that even in the future, God intends to return things to this peaceable kingdom where humans and animals live in peace and eat *only* plants. This kingdom is a restoration back to God's original intent of a harmless existence of companionship between humans and animals. You can do your part to at least restore God's perfect will in your life and make things on earth as they are in heaven for you by becoming a Christian vegan.

If you have done so, please contact me on my website at https://www.ChristianVeganism.com. I can send you a resource sheet of simple ways you can make your life vegan immediately and not have to worry about giving up the tastes that you enjoy or the quality of clothing that you wear. Vegan versions of foods, clothing, and other products far exceed the quality of the inferior animal-based versions. It is a very simple step to go vegan. Please do not let people tell you that you need to transition or take baby steps. You would not transition from any other harmful behavior you have realized was not God's will for you to partake of, rather you would give it up and start doing the right thing immediately.

James 4:17
17 Therefore to him that knoweth to do good,

and doeth *it* not, to him it is sin.

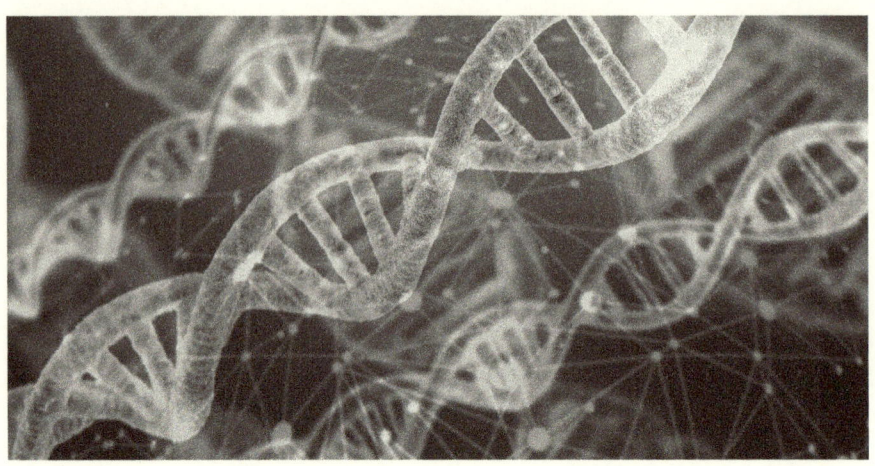

Chapter 5
What About My Health?

It is strange to see otherwise thoughtful people thoughtlessly repeating the propaganda of the meat, dairy, and egg industry. There is universal agreement about the health benefits of being vegan among thousands of studies investigating the health outcomes of hundreds of thousands of people. Only those completely removed from the massive amounts of data from the recent decades would hold to the old errors about needing to eat meat, dairy, or eggs for health.

In its annual meeting on June 14, 2017, the American Medical Association (AMA) House of Delegates, which represents more than 200,000 physician members, issued a resolution stating:

> "The American Medical Association hereby call on U.S. hospitals to improve the health of patients, staff, and visitors by (1) providing a variety of healthful food, including plant-based meals and meals that are low in fat, sodium,

and added sugars, (2) eliminating processed meats from menus, and (3) providing and promoting healthful beverages."

Another physicians group, the American Dietetic Association, noted in their position paper:

"It is the position of the American Dietetic Association that appropriately planned vegetarian diets, including total vegetarian or vegan diets, are healthful, nutritionally adequate, and may provide health benefits in the prevention and treatment of certain diseases. Well-planned vegetarian diets are appropriate for individuals during all stages of the life cycle, including pregnancy, lactation, infancy, childhood, and adolescence, and for athletes." (Source: https://www.ncbi.nlm.nih.gov/pubmed/19 562864)

From children to adults, all stages of the life cycle, a vegan diet is "healthful, nutritionally adequate, and may provide health benefits in the prevention and treatment of certain diseases." It is worth noting the phrase "appropriately planned" because one could technically eat vegan cookies all day and be eating a plant-based diet. The vegan cookie diet would obviously not be an "appropriately planned" vegan diet.

I am not picking on vegan cookies, and I will sometimes enjoy an occasional treat of a vegan cookie that you can see at https://ChristianVeganism.com/links/cookie every once in a while. I mention vegan cookies because I have heard non-vegans make absurd arguments using this line of illogic. No vegan is advocating for people to go on a processed food/junk food vegan diet. We encourage a healthy diet with plenty of fresh fruits and vegetables, legumes, and clean water.

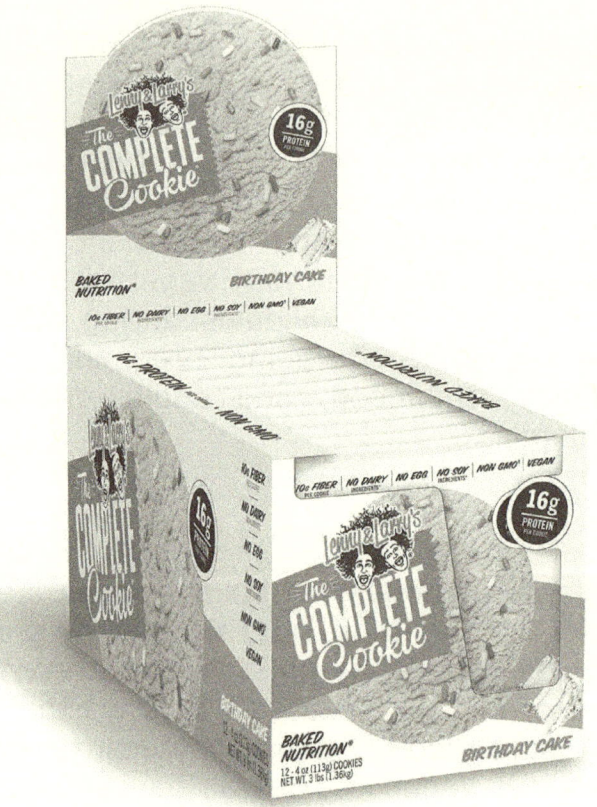

A delicious vegan cookie, no doubt, but it should not be the bulk of your diet!

When you hear of "vegans" who stopped being vegan for "health reasons," they are either lying about their actual diet or were eating processed foods all day. No one, vegan or not, reasonably thinks that eating processed foods is the best thing for your health, whether the processed food is vegan or not. There is simply no health benefit to eating animal flesh, drinking milk intended for other mammal's babies (or products made from it like butter and cheese), or eating the menstrual discharge of fowls (i.e. eggs).

The simple reality is that if you genuinely care about your health, then veganism is the only legitimate option for you because it is the most healthful diet and lifestyle that there is. I do not believe that your main reason for being a vegan should be health, as the moral imperative to be compassionate to other beings and the spiritual duty to best honor God with your life are more impactful reasons. With that having been said, the healthfulness of veganism is just another excellent benefit that you reap from doing the right thing and becoming a Christian vegan.

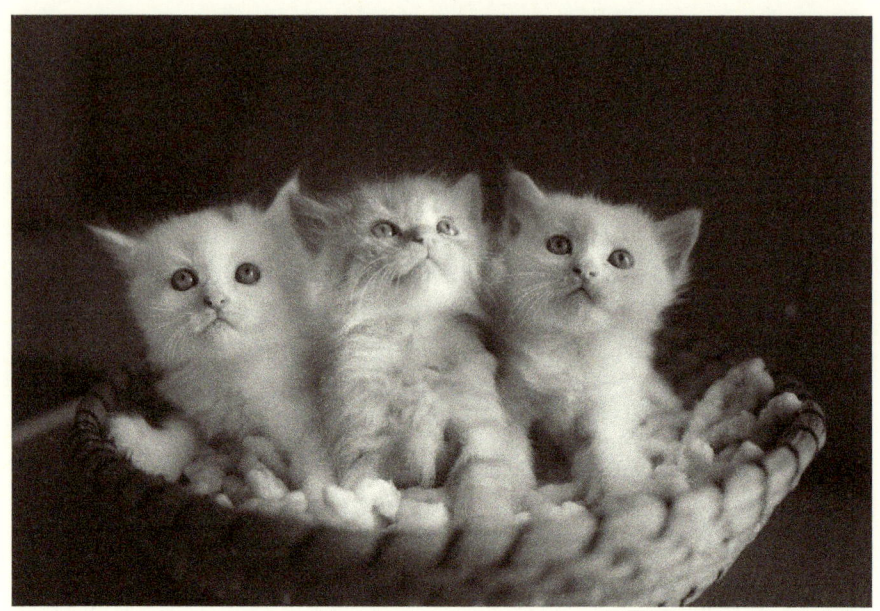

Chapter 6
Hear The Conclusion Of The Whole Matter

It is my prayer that this book has been used by the Spirit of Grace to enlighten the eyes of your understanding regarding the importance of following the Christian vegan lifestyle. I know that you may have many questions about certain verses of Scripture, teachings in Christendom, and other things that come to mind. As I mentioned in the Introduction, I have answered those questions and dealt with all the main passages of Scripture that people commonly bring up when trying to understand veganism from a Christian point of view in my book "Why Every Christian Should Be A Vegan." You can get it at https://www.ChristianVeganism.com

I am here to help you and hope that you will choose to have your life be one of peace, compassion, and love by becoming a Christian vegan. If you have any questions, need prayer, or want to learn more about Christian Veganism, please go to https://www.ChristianVeganism.com.

GO VEGAN

COMPASSION

NONVIOLENCE

FOR THE ANIMALS

FOR THE PLANET

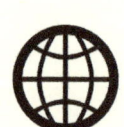

FOR THE PEOPLE

MAKE A DIFFERENCE!

GET THIS BOOK FOR YOUR FRIENDS AND FAMILY!

This book is great for church or study groups to go through together. It also serves as a great tool to help Christians who may not be vegans or vegans who may not be Christians. I encourage you to get this book into the hands of as many as will read it. I truly want to get this important book into as many hands as possible. Please go and sign up for my newsletter and you will get discounts and coupons for orders of two or more copies of the print version of this book: https://www.ChristianVeganism.com

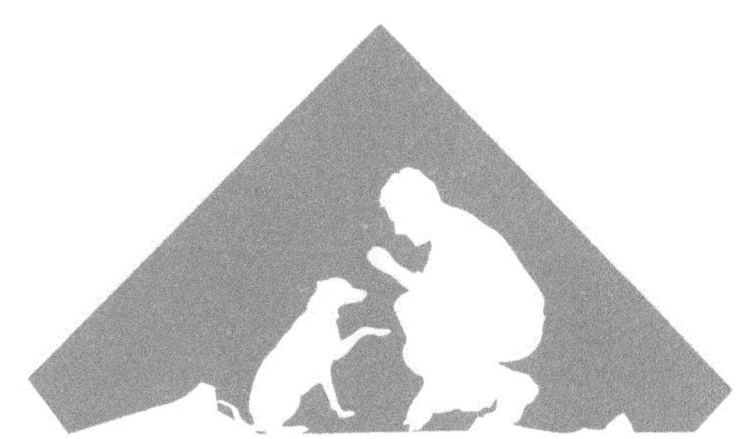

ChristianVeganism.com

Get the 400+ Page Book "Why Every Christian Should Be A Vegan" at
https://www.ChristianVeganism.com

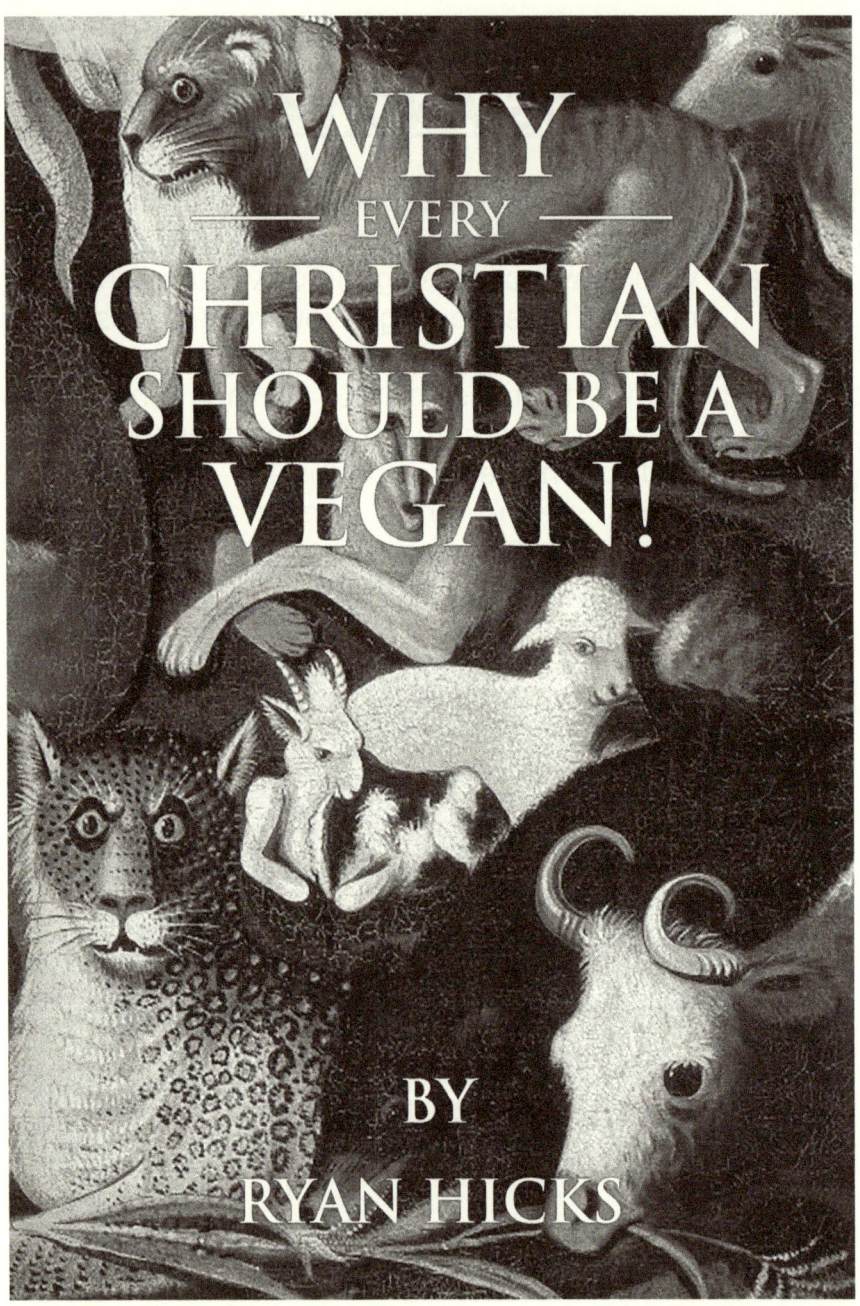

WHY
EVERY
CHRISTIAN
SHOULD BE A
VEGAN!

BY

RYAN HICKS

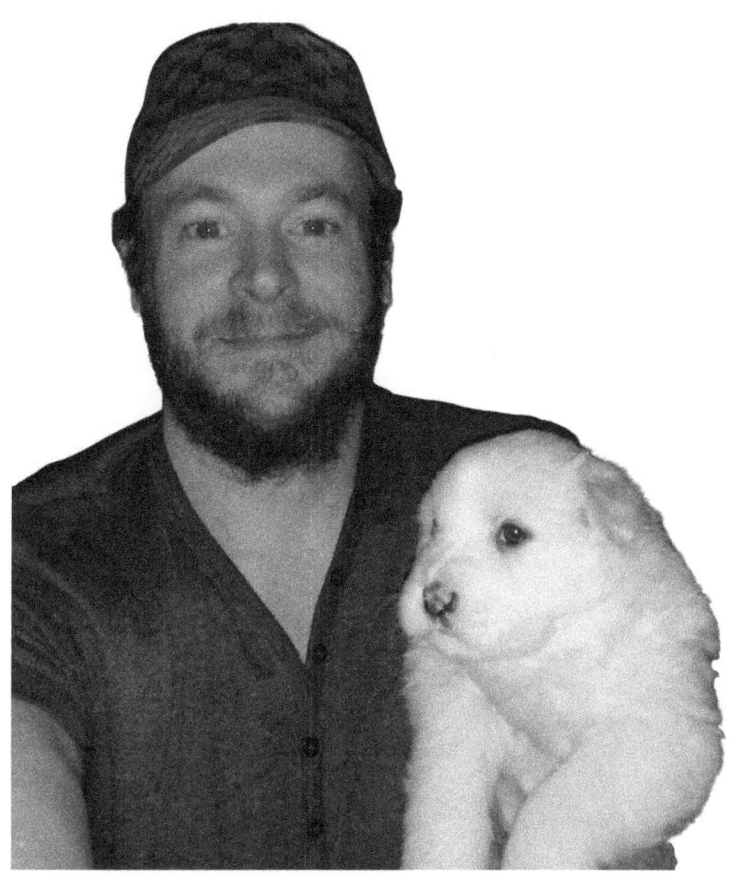

About The Author: I did not grow up in a vegetarian or vegan household. I did not personally know any vegans or watch any films on the virtues of veganism, and yet I still chose to become a vegan after being a life-long meat-eater. My book "Why Every Christian Should Be A Vegan" is the book that I wish I was given when I first started following Jesus. Had I been shown the ways of our compassionate Master towards animals then I would have certainly become a vegan much sooner. It is my faith-filled prayer that you will read this book and see the Christian way of mercy, peace, and love! My business and success related web site is https://www.TaughtToProfit.com